IT'S HARD —— TO —— GET FAT EATING SALADS

LANNY MORTON

It's Hard To Get Fat Eating Salads
Lanny Morton

ISBN-13: 978-0692117354 (Custom Universal)
ISBN-10: 0692117350

Interior design by Mariana Vidakovics De Victor

Contents

Introduction

This book is the equivalent of putting vitamins in the ice cream. What do I mean by that? What is in this book really works but let's face it, reading about crap like this is very boring.

I wrote this for those of you, like me, that are ADD and want to get results fast.

Warning: This book is offensive and has very bad language and probably should not be read by anyone, ever.. If this offends you, you were warned. I don't want to hear any whining about it.

If this book offends you, you are probably overweight and should take that pissed off energy and get off your ass and do something. Being overweight shortens your life, so doing nothing about your fat ass is literally possibly killing you.

Chapter 1

IT'S IN A BAG OR A BOX, WHAT SHOULD I DO?

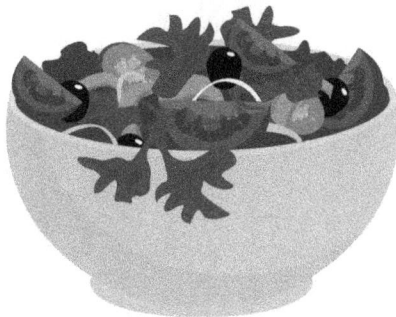

When Considering food
from a bag or a box,
Eat a fucking salad..

DO NOT EAT
Processed Foods!

Chapter 2

SHOULD I EAT RED MEAT?

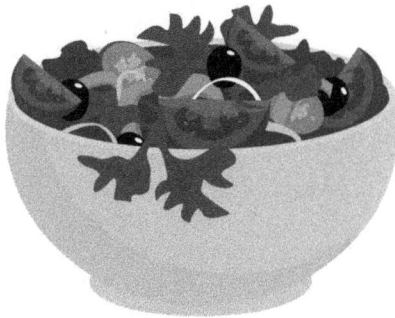

DO NOT EAT
Red Meat,

Eat a f*cking
salad instead

Chapter 3

DESSERT SOUNDS GOOD!

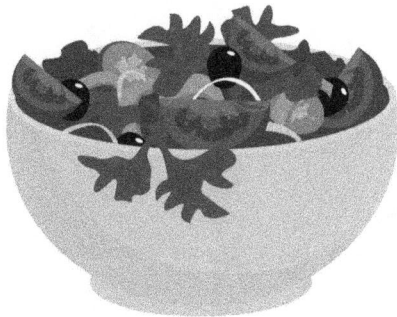

DO NOT EAT
Dessert,

have some more
f*cking salad…

Chapter 4

WHAT ABOUT BREAD? AND OTHER WHITE FLOUR PRODUCTS?

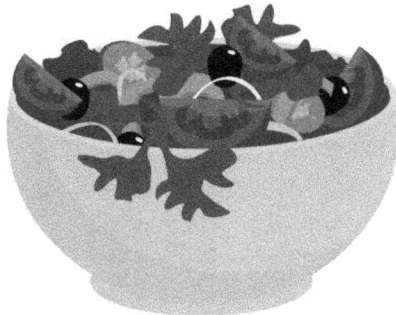

DO NOT EAT
White flour products

and lay off the bread,
and you guessed it,
eat a f*cking salad instead.

Chapter 5

IS BROCCOLI OR KALE GOOD FOR ME?

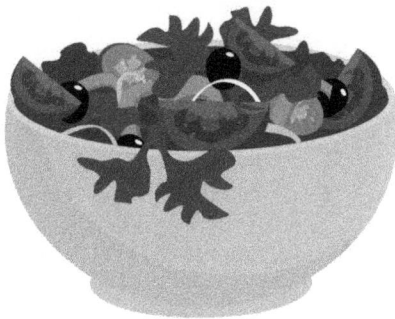

YES

Chapter 6

I ONLY WANT TO EXERCISE FOR 5 MINUTES A DAY BECAUSE I AM LAZY AS F*CK

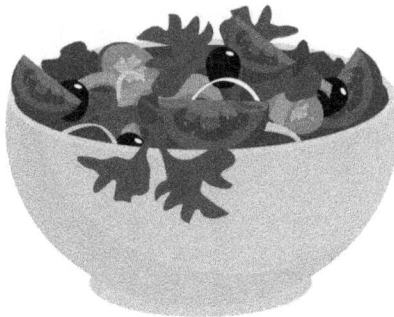

OK you lazy bastard,

you can either do **5 minutes** of kettlebell deadlifts or run uphill for **5 minutes**.

Either of them will drastically increase your resting calories burned.

Chapter 7

SHOULD I STAY AWAKE ALL NIGHT?

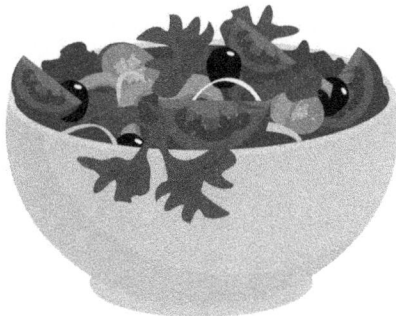

NO,

good sleep helps you lose weight dumbass.

Chapter 8

I AM VERY HUNGRY AND FAST FOOD LOOKS REALLY CONVENIENT

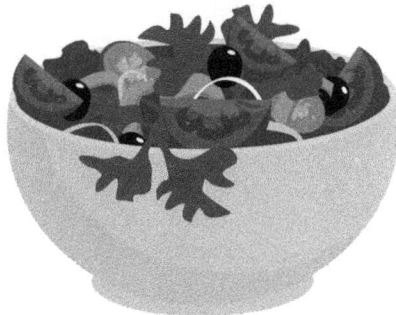

DON'T DO IT.

Go to a grocery store and
use the Salad Bar

Pro Tip:

Keep healthy snacks or food
with you at all times..

Chapter 9

SHOULD I DRINK A 6 PACK OF BEER EVERY NIGHT?

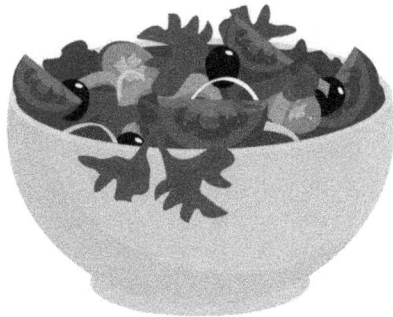

NO...

JACKASS...

Chapter 10

IS PROCESSED SUGAR GOOD FOR ME?

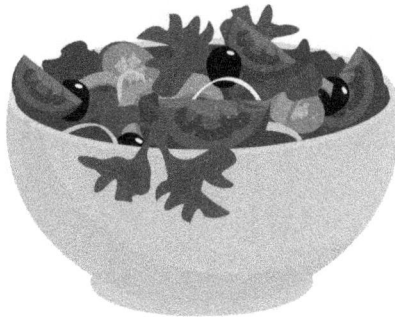

No, Jackwagon,

avoid sugar of any kind,
especially processed.

Chapter 11

HOW LONG WILL IT TAKE TO LOSE WEIGHT FOLLOWING THIS COMPLEX BOOK?

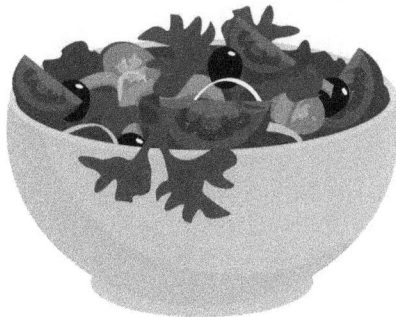

You should lose about
10 POUNDS
in your first month
and probably
ANOTHER 10
in month 2.

Chapter 12

WHAT HAPPENS
IF I SCREW UP?

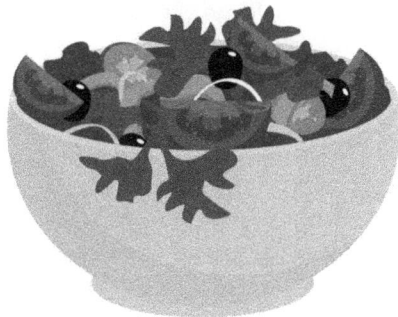

Let it go.

Make the next right decision.

Resentment of yourself or others will keep you a fat ass..

And eat another f*ckng salad…

Chapter 13

SHOULD I EAT FOOD AFTER 7PM?

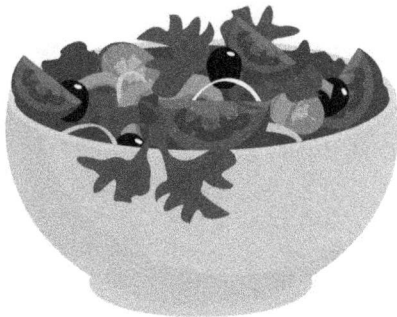

NO

Chapter 14

SHOULD MY POOP LOOK LIKE A MARBLE?

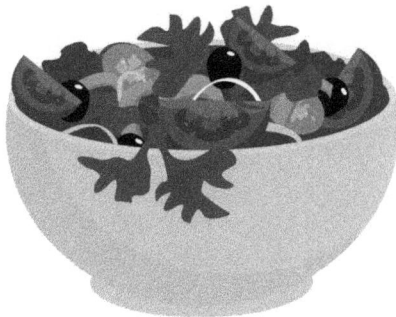

No,

A majestic, beautiful, healthy dump should not look like a marble or a bunch of marbles stuck together. It should come out smooth and in the shape of your colon. If you feel like you are giving birth and it tears your asshole as it comes out,

you probably need to eat a fucking salad.

Chapter 15

EATING OUT

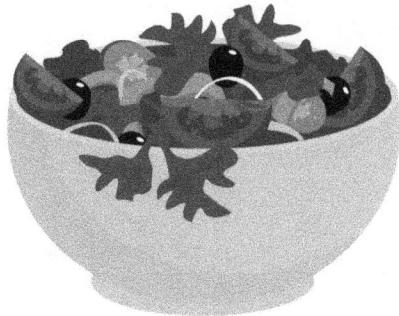

If you want to get rid of a few extra pounds, the only Eating Out you should be doing should be on your wife or girlfriend or a girl that's a friend that needs an attitude adjustment.

Have you ever noticed that the salads at restaurants have as many calories as ordering a steak?

You just don't know what people in restaurants are putting in your food.

Pro Tip:

If you have to eat out at a restaurant, you can't go wrong ordering an unseasoned chicken breast and unseasoned broccoli.

Pro Tip #2:

When Eating Out, don't stop doing what's working. When you change it up, you lose momentum and takes longer to get results.

Chapter 16

DAIRY PRODUCTS

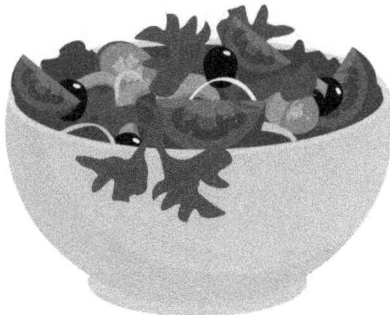

Milk is for baby cows. Not for people.

The Dairy industry spends over $6 million a year on lobbyists. Do you think they have to spend all that money because dairy products are good for you?

Last year, The Dairy industry spent over $1 Billion on advertising attempting to convince you that dairy is good for you and you should drink it.

Fun Fact: The World Health organization does not have dairy on their food pyramid.

Another Fun Fact: The US Dept. Of Agriculture has it on there because of lobbyists.

Triple Fun Fact: The myth that dairy is good for your bones isn't true.

Remember,
when you drink milk,
you are basically sucking on
a cow's tit. Instead of doing
that, go suck on the tit of
your significant other. It's
more fun and better for you.

Chapter 17

WHERE DO I GO FOR MORE SUPER VALUABLE INFORMATION LIKE THIS?

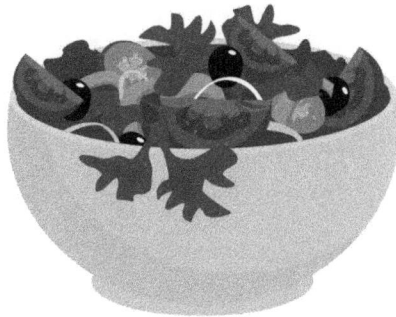

If you would like more ridiculously simple but highly effective advice, I have a completely free 90 day challenge that will help you make more money, be healthy, and have great relationships.

People have said it was life changing for them, but I don't believe them.

Set up your free account [1]
https://www.motivation.net/free

---

1 https://www.motivation.net/new-account-setup-for-90-day-challenge

I am not a doctor or a dietician.

The information I provide is based on my personal experience of taking the best information from several very expensive, super fancy health facilities and boiling down to something that is simple and hopefully entertaining.

I was able to get rid of 26 pounds in two months doing this. (And Exercise)

Any recommendations I may make about exercise, nutrition or lifestyle, or information provided to you in this book **should be discussed between you and your doctor** because working out involves risks. The information you receive in this book does not take the place of professional medical advice

Before starting any new diet and exercise program please check with your doctor and clear any exercise and/or diet changes with them before beginning.

motivation.net ™

"Ignite your burning desire to achieve your dreams"

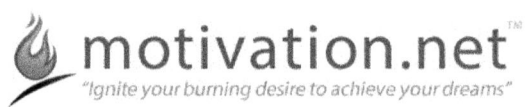

www.ingramcontent.com/pod-product-compliance
Lightning Source LLC
Chambersburg PA
CBHW022127280326
41933CB00007B/584